THE WORLD'S SIMPLEST KETO DIET BOOK

Healthy Eating that Tastes Delicious with an Easy-to-Follow 30-Day Meal Plan

NICHOLAS R. GARDNER

ISBN – 9798801173092

TABLE OF CONTENTS

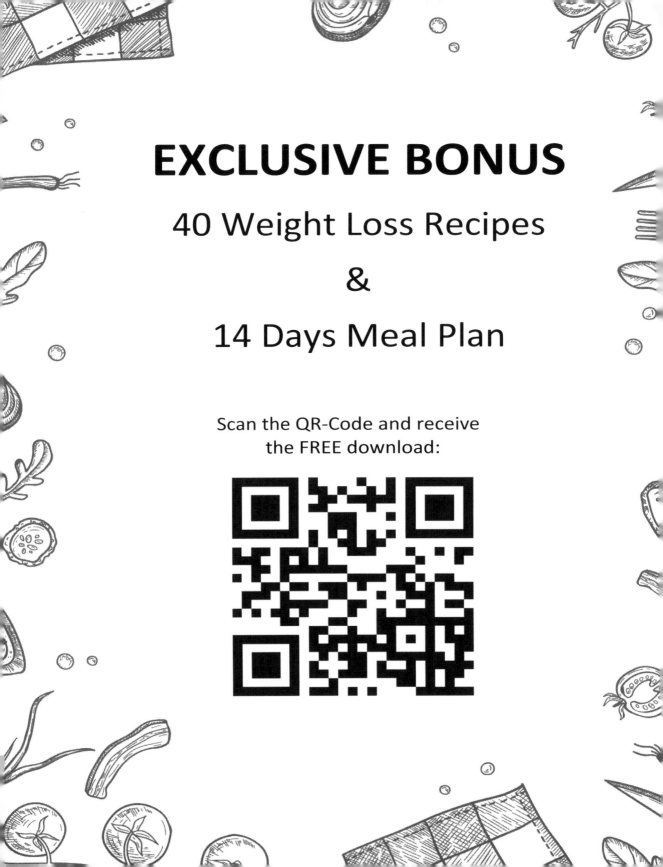

EXCLUSIVE BONUS

40 Weight Loss Recipes

&

14 Days Meal Plan

Scan the QR-Code and receive
the FREE download:

Keto 101

Food is fuel- we all know that right? This fuel for the majority of people is primarily made up of carbohydrates- grains, fruit, sugar, wheat etc. Carbohydrates are broken down into glucose and metabolised for energy. The issue with this 'traditional' energy source is that when the glucose/energy isn't used it is stored in the body as fat, and this fat can be difficult to get rid of.

The keto diet avoids excess fat storage. This low-carb high-fat diet designed for rapid, sustainable weight loss and increased physical functioning. The diet works by inducing a metabolic state known as ketosis through the restriction of carbohydrates... and our bodies are clever- if there aren't carbohydrates for fuel what can be used instead?

This is when ketosis comes in. Restriction of carbohydrates induces ketosis to meet our energy needs. When carbohydrates aren't available our bodies release chemical compounds called ketones into our blood stream, and these little miracles work to transform fat into energy rather than carbohydrates. Both dietary and bodily fat are targeted as energy sources by ketones.

This is why the keto diet is high-fat – fat is necessary to provide an energy source whilst maintaining normal levels of cognitive functioning. Carbohydrates are replaced by fat within your diet, and so it is recommended to have 70%-80% of your overall calorific intake coming from fat sources.

Once the restriction of carbohydrates has begun the body will naturally enter a stage of ketosis after 3-5 days (if consuming less than 50g of carbohydrates per day). Net carbs (digestible carbohydrates) are counted on the keto diet instead of calories, with emphasis being on micro and macro nutrients rather than the classic 'low-fat' or 'low-calorie' emphasis that most diets insist upon.

Everyone's keto diet plan is different depending upon your age, current weight, height, gender, energy levels, and so on, so it is recommended that you use an online calculator tool to work out the most effective diet plan for your individual needs and goals.

Benefits of the keto diet include:

- ✓ Sustainable weight loss
- ✓ Increased energy
- ✓ Increased mental functioning- focus, concentration, and overall clarity
- ✓ Maintaining muscle mass
- ✓ Heightened physical performance
- ✓ Improved skin condition, in particular the effects of acne
- ✓ Settling of persistent stomach issues, such as IBS, gas, and cramping
- ✓ Appetite regulator and feelings of increased satiety
- ✓ Reduced cravings for high carbohydrate foods

Keto isn't magic- a healthy overall lifestyle is always recommended- but it is pretty spectacular! Whole communities have sprung up in awe of this diet, and many lives have been changed for the better. As either a short- or long-term solution the keto diet offers a delicious, sustainable diet with benefits reaching far beyond losing a few pounds. Begin your keto lifestyle today and see what transformations you can achieve!

Breakfast

Mushroom Baked Eggs

Serves	4
Carbohydrates	2g
Protein	6.7g
Fat	5.6g
Calories	86

INGREDIENTS

- 4 Portobello mushrooms, washed and destalked
- 1 tsp olive oil
- 2 tsp garlic, minced
- 4 eggs
- 1 tsp fresh thyme leaves
- Rocket or spinach to serve
- Salt and pepper to taste

DIRECTIONS

1. Begin by preheating your oven to 200C // 400F. Arrange your mushrooms, facing upwards, on a baking tray before brushing over your olive oil and dividing your minced garlic between the mushrooms. Place your mushrooms in the oven to bake for 20 minutes.

2. After 20 minutes remove your mushrooms from the oven. Crack an egg into each mushroom then sprinkle over your thyme. Return the mushrooms to the oven for another 10-15 minutes, or until the whites are cooked through and the yolks are to your liking.

Remove the mushrooms from the oven and transfer to plates. Garnish with rocket or spinach leaves to serve.

Herby Frittata

Serves	4
Carbohydrates	2.5g
Protein	7.9g
Fat	11.9g
Calories	114

INGREDIENTS

- 1 tbsp olive oil
- 4 eggs
- ½ tsp turmeric
- ½ tsp cumin
- 2 tsp fresh coriander, finely chopped
- 2 tsp fresh basil, finely chopped
- 4 spring onions, finely sliced
- 2 tbsp walnuts, roughly chopped
- 30g // 1oz. crumbled feta, plus extra to serve
- Salt and pepper to taste
- Leafy greens to serve

DIRECTIONS

1. Begin by setting your grill to 'high' and leaving to heat, and while the grill heats use your oil to grease a small frying pan. In a small bowl whisk together your eggs, turmeric, cumin, coriander, basil, spring onions, and season with salt and pepper. Pour this egg mixture into your frying pan.
2. Cook your eggs over a medium heat, not stirring or disrupting the mix too much. After 10 minutes, or once your eggs are almost cooked through, turn off the heat and sprinkle over your walnuts and feta. Transfer the frying pan and mixture to your heated grill and cook for a further 2 minutes.

Serve your frittata immediately, topped with extra feta and accompanied by leafy greens.

Egg and Asparagus Soldiers

Serves	2
Carbohydrates	8.3g
Protein	9.9g
Fat	7g
Calories	124

INGREDIENTS

- 2 eggs
- 16 asparagus spears
- 1 tsp olive oil
- ½ tsp smoked paprika
- Pinch of chilli powder

DIRECTIONS

1. Bring a large saucepan of salted water to the boil. Drop in your asparagus spears and cook for 3-5 minutes, or until tender but retaining some bite. While the asparagus cooks, heat your oil in a medium saucepan over a high heat.

2. When your asparagus are cooked place your eggs into the boiling water and remove your asparagus spears with a slotted spoon. Immediately place the spears into your frying pan, then sprinkle over your paprika and chilli powder and flash fry for 1-2 minutes. Divide between 2 plates once fried.

3. By this time, your eggs should be soft boiled – 3-4 minutes. Remove your eggs from the water and transfer each to an egg cup. Cut the top off each egg and serve immediately.

Egg and Feta Hash

Serves	2
Carbohydrates	12.9g
Protein	16.7g
Fat	27.4g
Calories	366

INGREDIENTS

- 2 tbsp coconut oil
- 2 button mushrooms, washed and sliced
- 6 cherry tomatoes, halved or quartered
- 2 spring onions, finely sliced
- 60g // 2oz. crumbled feta
- 3 eggs
- 2 tsp chives, roughly chopped
- 2 generous handfuls of spinach
- Salt and pepper to taste

DIRECTIONS

1. Heat your coconut oil in a medium frying pan over a low heat. Once the oil is melted add your mushrooms, tomatoes, and spring onions, and sauté for 3-5 minutes or until softened. Sprinkle over your feta and cook for a further minute.

2. In a separate bowl whisk your eggs until light and fluffy before adding your chives, and seasoning with salt and pepper. Whisk to combine everything before pouring the egg mixture into your frying pan.

Continue to whisk the mixture to fully combine all the ingredients and scramble your eggs. Once the eggs are scrambled to your liking divide the mixture between 2 bowls. Serve accompanied by a handful of spinach.

Bacon Breakfast Tacos

Serves	4
Carbohydrates	7.6g
Protein	31.3g
Fat	73.4g
Calories	815

INGREDIENTS

- 16 rashers of bacon
- 4 eggs
- 1 tbsp full cream milk
- 1 tbsp salted butter
- 1 tbsp smoked paprika
- 120g // 4oz. grated cheddar
- 1 avocado, diced
- Salt and pepper to taste

DIRECTIONS

1. Begin by preheating your oven to 200C // 400F and lining a large baking tray with foil or greaseproof paper. Cut each bacon rasher in half and divide the rasher between 4 – this means 4 full rasher, or 8 halved rashers each.

2. Weave your rashers to create a 4x4 square. Repeat this until you have 4 lattices arranged on your baking tray. Place your bacon into the oven and bake for 25-30 minutes, or until it is crispy and cooked. Once cooked remove from the oven and cut each lattice into a circle.

3. Set the bacon aside while you cook your scrambled eggs. Crack your eggs into a small saucepan and add in your milk, butter, and paprika. Season with salt and pepper, then whisk to combine. Turn the heat to medium and continue whisking until the eggs are scrambled to your liking, then remove from the heat.

Serve your tacos by dividing your eggs between the bacon rounds. Sprinkle over your cheese and diced avocado, before folding in half to create a taco and eating immediately.

Cauliflower Eggs Benedict

Serves	2
Carbohydrates	8.3g
Protein	46.4g
Fat	69.1g
Calories	844

INGREDIENTS

- ½ a large head of cauliflower
- 1 egg
- 235g // 4oz. grated cheddar
- 1 tbsp olive oil
- 4 egg yolks
- 2 tbsp lemon juice
- 6 ½ tbsp butter, melted
- 2 poached eggs
- Fresh chopped chives to serve
- Salt and pepper to taste

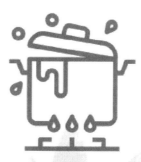

DIRECTIONS

1. Begin by making your cauliflower crumpets. Do this by grating your cauliflower into a large mixing bowl containing your egg and cheddar. Season the mix with salt and pepper before mixing everything together with a wooden spoon. Once mixed divide the mixture into two and shape each half into a patty.

2. Heat your olive oil over a high heat in a medium frying pan. Add your patties to the heated oil and fry for 5 minutes each side, or until golden brown and crispy. Transfer to a paper towel lined plate and set aside.

3. Make your hollandaise sauce by first placing a glass bowl over a saucepan of simmering water. Add your egg yolks and lemon juice to the bowl, and whisk until the yolks lighten in colour. Pour in your melted butter as a steady trickle, whisking constantly so ensure all the butter combines as it is poured in. Continue to whisk as you season with salt and pepper, then remove from the heat.

Assemble your Benedict by layering a poached egg on top of your warm cauliflower patty. Drizzle over your benedict sauce and top with fresh chives to serve.

Everything Bagels

Serves	8
Carbohydrates	2.2g
Protein	10.3g
Fat	16.6g
Calories	210

INGREDIENTS

- 240g // 16oz. grated mozzarella
- 5 tbsp cream cheese
- 2 large eggs (+ 1 lightly beaten for an egg wash)
- 200g // 2 c almond flour
- 3 tsp baking powder
- 4 tbsp 'everything bagel' seed mix or seasoning

DIRECTIONS

1. Begin by preheating your oven to 200C // 400F, and line 2 medium baking trays with parchment paper.

2. Place your grated mozzarella and cream cheese into a large, microwave safe bowl, and stir to roughly combine. Place into the microwave and heat on high for 30 second intervals, stirring in between. Continue until everything is melted and combined- roughly 2 minutes. Whilst the mixture heats, pour your almond flour and baking powder into a large bowl and whisk to combine.

3. Spoon your cheese mixture into your flour and add your 2 eggs. Mix with a wooden spoon or your hands until everything is thoroughly combined, then divide this mixture into 8 portions. Roll each portion into a ball, then push your thumb through the centre of each to create a bagel shape.

4. Transfer your bagels onto the prepared baking trays, then brush each with your egg wash and top with 'everything bagel' mix. Place into the preheated oven and bake for 20-25 minutes, or until golden brown with a firm exterior and cooked through.

Allow your bagels to cool slightly before topping with your favourite fillings to serving.

Stuffed Tomatoes

Serves	2
Carbohydrates	4.9g
Protein	22.9g
Fat	21.6g
Calories	301

INGREDIENTS

- 2 large beef tomatoes
- 1 tbsp olive oil
- 2 eggs
- 2 tbsp fresh basil, finely chopped
- 4 tbsp grated mozzarella
- Salt and pepper to taste

DIRECTIONS

1. Begin by preheating your oven to 200C // 400F and lining a small baking tray with foil or greaseproof paper. Slice the tops off your tomatoes and remove the seeds and flesh with a spoon or knife. Brush over your olive oil before placing the tomatoes into the oven to bake for 10 minutes.

2. After 10 minutes remove your tomatoes from the oven. Crack an egg into both hollows before seasoning with salt and pepper and sprinkling over your fresh basil. Return the oven to bake for a further 10-15 minutes.

After 10-15 minutes, or once the whites are cooked through and the yolks are to your liking, remove your tomatoes from the oven and sprinkle over your grated mozzarella to serve.

Egg and Ham Wrap

Serves	2
Carbohydrates	9.7g
Protein	28.3g
Fat	17g
Calories	314

INGREDIENTS

- 4 eggs
- 1 tbsp water
- 1 tsp cornflour
- 1 tsp olive oil
- 85g // 12oz. grated cheddar

- 2 slices ham
- Salt and pepper to taste
- 4 cherry tomatoes to serve
- Spinach to serve

DIRECTIONS

1. Place the cornflour and water into a small mixing bowl and whisk until a thick paste forms. Add in your eggs and salt and continue to whisk until it is fully combined, light, and fluffy.

2. Heat your oil in a medium sized pan before pouring in your egg mixture. Spread the mixture to form a thin layer over the whole pan. Fry for 2-4 minutes on each side, or until the egg is cooked and the edges are browned.

Add your ham and cheese and cover your pan with a lid for 1 minute to melt the cheese. Repeat this process, and once both wraps are cooked roll them into a wrap shape and serve immediately, accompanied by your cherry tomatoes and spinach.

Savoury Cauliflower Waffles

Serves	3
Carbohydrates	13.4g
Protein	25.7g
Fat	23.1g
Calories	378

INGREDIENTS

- ½ a large cauliflower head
- 300g // 10oz. grated mozzarella
- 55g // 2oz. grated parmesan
- 3 eggs
- 30g // ¼ c cornflour
- 1 tbsp chilli sauce
- Salt and pepper to taste
- 3 fried eggs to serve
- ½ avocado to serve

DIRECTIONS

1. Begin by turning your waffle iron to high and leaving it to heat up. As it heats, grate your cauliflower into a large mixing bowl before adding in your mozzarella, parmesan, eggs, cornflour, chilli sauce, and seasoning. Beat everything together to form a thick batter.

2. Pour your batter into your heated waffle iron, spreading the mixture into the corners to ensure even cooking. Cook the waffle for 5-7 minutes, or until golden brown and crispy.

Transfer your waffle to a plate and serve with sliced avocado and a fried egg.

Pumpkin Pancakes

Serves	2
Carbohydrates	7.2g
Protein	11.4g
Fat	28.3g
Calories	342

INGREDIENTS

- 60g // 2oz. almond flour
- ¼ tsp baking powder
- ½ tsp salt
- 1 tbsp cinnamon
- 1 tsp nutmeg
- 1 tsp ground ginger
- ½ tsp ground cloves
- ½ tsp allspice
- 2 eggs, separated
- 60ml // ¼ c double cream
- 60ml // ¼ c pumpkin puree
- 1 tsp butter
- Full fat Greek yoghurt to serve

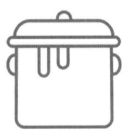

DIRECTIONS

1. Sift your almond flour, baking powder, salt, cinnamon, nutmeg, ginger, cloves, and allspice into a large mixing bowl. In a separate bowl whisk together your egg yolks, double cream, and pumpkin puree. Once fully combined add this to your dry ingredients, then whisk everything until the mixture is smooth.

2. Taking a separate bowl, clean electric whisk, beat your egg whites into stiff peaks. Gently fold your egg whites into the batter, being careful to keep in as much air as possible.

Melt your butter in a medium frying pan over a high heat. Once the butter has melted, spoon in your pancake batter, using 4 tbsp // ¼ c of batter per pancake. Cook the pancakes for around 2 minutes per side, or until beginning to brown. Once cooked transfer the pancakes to plates and top with a dollop of Greek yoghurt to serve.

Berry Blast Smoothie

Serves	2
Carbohydrates	10.5g
Protein	6.5g
Fat	14.3g
Calories	215

INGREDIENTS

- ½ avocado
- 30g // 1 c spinach
- 150g // 1 c blackberries
- 250ml // 1 c full cream milk
- 500ml // 2 c ice

DIRECTIONS

Place all the ingredients into a blender and blend on high until a thick and creamy liquid has formed. Divide between 2 cups and serve.

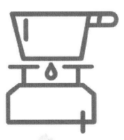

Granola

Serves	10
Carbohydrates	3.4g
Protein	8.7g
Fat	34.6g
Calories	364

INGREDIENTS

- 150g // 1 c almonds, roughly chopped
- 150g // 1 c walnuts, roughly chopped
- 150g // 1 c coconut flakes/chunks
- 2 tbsp sesame seeds
- 2 tbsp flax seeds
- 2 tbsp chia seeds
- 1 ½ tsp cinnamon
- ½ tsp ground clove
- ½ tsp ground ginger
- 1 tsp vanilla extract
- Pinch of salt
- 1 egg white
- 120ml // ¼ c coconut oil, melted

DIRECTIONS

1. Begin by preheating your oven to 180C // 350F, and line or grease a large baking tray. In a large mixing bowl combine all your dry ingredients.
2. In a separate bowl whisk the egg white until it begins to thicken, then stir in melted coconut oil. Add the egg white and melted coconut oil to your dry mix.
3. Combine your wet and dry ingredients, stirring thoroughly to ensure everything is coated, then pour onto your prepared pan and flatten.

Bake for 10 minutes, stir, and then return to the oven for a further 10-15 minutes. Cool the granola on the pan before transferring to an airtight container.

Banana Waffles

Serves	4
Carbohydrates	11.3g
Protein	10.6g
Fat	23.4g
Calories	299

INGREDIENTS

- 1 banana, mashed
- 4 eggs
- 100g // ¾ c almond flour
- 175ml // ¾ c coconut milk
- 1 tbsp ground psyllium husk powder
- 1 tsp baking powder
- ½ tsp vanilla extract
- Pinch of salt

DIRECTIONS

1. Begin by turning on your waffle iron and leaving it to heat. In a medium mixing bowl use a wooden spoon to beat together eggs, coconut milk, vanilla extract, and mashed banana until smooth.

2. In a separate bowl sieve the almond flour, psyllium husk powder, baking powder, and salt together, then fold this mix into your wet ingredients- be careful to keep as much air as possible. Allow the mixture to sit for 15-20 minutes.

3. Spoon your mixture into your preheated waffle iron and cook for 6 minutes, or until golden brown and crispy.

Serve with cream, butter, hazelnut spread, or whatever else takes your fancy.

Mains

Mushroom Soup

Serves	4
Carbohydrates	8.2g
Protein	5.8g
Fat	12.1g
Calories	166

INGREDIENTS

- 3 tbsp butter
- 1 brown onion, diced
- 1 tbsp garlic, minced
- 500g // 4 c mushrooms, washed and finely chopped
- 1 tbsp plain flour
- 1l // 4 c vegetable stock
- 1 bay leaf
- 2 tbsp double cream
- 1 tbsp dried parsley

DIRECTIONS

1. In a large heavy bottomed pan melt your butter over a medium heat. Add in your onion and garlic and sauté until softened. Add mushrooms to the pan and cook for a further 3-5 minutes, or until your mushrooms are softened, but still retaining a little bite.

2. Sift over your flour and stir to combine before pouring in your vegetable stock and bay leaf, and bringing the mix to a simmer.

3. Leave the soup to simmer for 10-15 minutes before removing the bay leaf and pouring the mix into a food processor. Add in your double cream and bay leaf, then blend to form a thick, creamy liquid.

4. Return your soup to the pan and heat. Ladle the hot soup into bowls and serve.

Celery Soup

Serves	4
Carbohydrates	3.5g
Protein	2g
Fat	8.1g
Calories	100

INGREDIENTS

- 2 tbsp olive oil
- 300g //10oz. celery, roughly chopped
- 1 tbsp garlic, minced
- 100g // 4oz. cauliflower, cut into florets
- 500ml // 2 c vegetable stocks
- 100ml // 2/3 c full cream milk
- Salt and pepper to taste

DIRECTIONS

1. Heat your oil in a large heavy bottomed pan, then pour in your celery, garlic, and cauliflower florets. Season with salt and pepper, then cook the vegetables for 10-15 minutes, or until softened and lightly coloured. Pour in your vegetable stock and bring the mixture to the boil.

2. Reduce the heat and leave the mixture to simmer for 15-20 minutes. Transfer the mix to a food processor, pouring in your milk before blending on high to form a thick, creamy liquid.

Return your soup to the pan and heat. Ladle the hot soup into bowls and serve.

Slow Cooker Prawn Soup

Serves	4
Carbohydrates	8.4g
Protein	28.2g
Fat	50.2g
Calories	593

INGREDIENTS

- 180g // 6.5oz. cauliflower, cut into florets
- 140g // 5oz. broccoli, cut into florets
- 110g // 4oz. turnip, diced
- 500ml // 2c double cream
- 1l // 4c fish stock
- 240g // 8.5oz. frozen prawn
- 110g // 4oz. frozen shrimp
- Salt and pepper to taste
- Drizzle of cream to serve

DIRECTIONS

1. Prepare your vegetables and place them into the bowl of your slow cooker, then pour over your double cream and fish stock. Stir to roughly combine then place the lid on your slow cooker and leave it on 'low' for 4.5 hours.

2. After 4.5 hours blend your mixture with a handheld blender or by transferring to a food processor. Add your frozen shrimp and prawns to the blended mix in the slow cooker. Season with salt and pepper, stir to roughly combine, then replace the lid of your slow cooker and leave to cook for a further 1-1.5 hours.

Once the prawns and shrimp are cooked and the soup is hot to your liking ladle it into bowls. Top with a drizzle of cream to serve.

Clam Chowder

Serves	4
Carbohydrates	3.2g
Protein	5.8g
Fat	18.4g
Calories	203

INGREDIENTS

- 6 tbsp butter
- 1 small white onion, sliced
- 230g // 8oz. cauliflower, cut into florets
- 500ml // 2c fish stock
- 500ml // 2c water
- 450g // 1lb. clams, still in shell
- 70g // 2.5oz. shelled clams
- Salt and pepper to taste
- Dried rosemary to serve
- Cream to serve

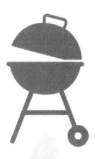

DIRECTIONS

1. Heat 2 tbsp of your butter in a large pot. Sauté your onions for 3-5 minutes, or until softened and translucent, then add in half of your cauliflower and cook for a further 3-5 minutes, or until beginning to soften.

2. Pour in your fish stock, water, and remaining butter. Stir to combine before bringing the mixture to a boil, then reducing the heat and leaving to simmer for 10-15 minutes. After 10-15 minutes transfer your mixture to a food processor and blend until smooth.

3. Return your blended mixture to the pot and pour in your remaining cauliflower florets and clams. Season with salt and pepper before heating to a simmer and leaving to cook for another 10 minutes.

Ladle your chowder into bowls and top with a sprinkling of dried rosemary and a drizzle of cream to serve.

Gazpacho

Serves	4
Carbohydrates	13.5g
Protein	3.5g
Fat	7.7g
Calories	141

INGREDIENTS

- 🍽 1kg // 2.2lb assorted tomatoes, roughly chopped
- 🍽 1 red bell pepper, roughly chopped
- 🍽 1 medium cucumber, peeled and diced
- 🍽 1 tbsp garlic, minced
- 🍽 1 medium red onion, finely diced
- 🍽 4 tbsp fresh basil, finely chopped
- 🍽 2 tbsp olive oil
- 🍽 Salt and pepper to taste

DIRECTIONS

1. Place your tomatoes, red pepper, cucumber, garlic, half of your onion, and half of your basil into a food processor. Blend on high until a thick, smooth mixture forms. Season with salt and pepper, then blend again to combine.

Ladle the gazpacho into bowls and serve topped with your remaining onion and basil, and with a drizzle of olive oil.

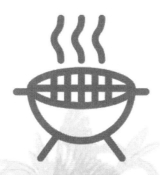

Thai Butternut Soup

Serves	4
Carbohydrates	12.8g
Protein	4.7g
Fat	32.6g
Calories	407

INGREDIENTS

- 1 medium butternut squash, peeled, deseeded, and roughly chopped
- 1 medium white onion, diced
- 1 tbsp coconut oil
- 4 tbsp red curry paste
- 2 tbsp fresh ginger, minced
- 4 tbsp garlic, minced
- 1 tsp turmeric
- 500ml // 2c vegetable stock
- 400ml // 14oz. coconut milk
- 1 tbsp dark soy sauce
- 1 tsp maple syrup
- 1 tbsp fresh lime juice
- Salt and pepper to taste

DIRECTIONS

1. Begin by preheating your oven to 180C // 350F and arranging your butternut and onion on a large baking tray. Pour over your coconut oil and red curry paste, then toss everything together before transferring to the oven to roast for 45-50 minutes, or until the butternut is softened.

2. Once the butternut has roasted transfer it to a food processor. Add in you ginger, garlic, turmeric, and vegetable stock, and blend until smooth. Pour the soup into a large heavy bottomed pan and heat. Once heated slowly pour your coconut milk into the soup, stirring continuously to ensure the milk is fully combined.

3. Heat for a further 5 minutes before adding in your soy sauce, maple syrup, and lime juice. Season with salt and pepper before ladling into bowls and serving immediately.

Cauliflower Steak

Serves	2
Carbohydrates	8.1g
Protein	4.2g
Fat	13.6g
Calories	178

INGREDIENTS

- 1 red pepper
- ½ tsp cumin
- 1 tsp smoked paprika
- 2 tbsp butter, melted
- 1 tsp capers
- 2 tsp red wine vinegar
- 1 small cauliflower head, halved
- 1 tbsp almonds, roughly chopped, to serve

DIRECTIONS

1. Begin by preheating your oven to 200C // 400F. Roughly chop your pepper and place it on a medium baking tray, then transfer to the oven to roast for 20-30 minutes, or until softened and browned.

2. Remove your pepper from the oven and transfer it to a small blender. Add your cumin, paprika, butter, capers, and red wine vinegar, and blend to form a paste. Arrange your cauliflower halves, flat side down, on your baking tray before covering with the red pepper paste.

Place your coated cauliflowers in the hot oven and leave to roast for 20-25 minutes, or until cooked through. Transfer to plates before sprinkling over your chopped almonds and serving.

Goats Cheese and Celery Boats

Serves	1
Carbohydrates	7.9g
Protein	28g
Fat	30.1g
Calories	421

INGREDIENTS

- 120g // 4oz. soft goats cheese
- 2 tbsp garlic, minced
- 1 tsp fresh basil, finely sliced
- 6 celery stalks, washed
- Salt and pepper to taste
- Fresh basil to serve

DIRECTIONS

1. Begin by preheating your oven to 180C // 350F. In a small bowl mix together your goats cheese, garlic, and basil, ensuring the herbs are evenly distributed.
2. Fill the hollows of your celery with the goats cheese and arrange the sticks on a baking tray. Season with salt and pepper before transferring to the oven and baking for 30-40 minutes, or until the celery is cooked but not wet.

Remove from the oven and transfer to plates. Top with more fresh basil and serve.

Greek Salad Slabs

Serves	4
Carbohydrates	9.1g
Protein	7.8g
Fat	41.7g
Calories	440

INGREDIENTS

DRESSING

- 🍽 120ml // ½ c olive oil
- 🍽 1 tbsp Dijon mustard
- 🍽 1 tbsp garlic, minced
- 🍽 1 tsp fresh basil, finely sliced
- 🍽 1 tsp dried oregano
- 🍽 60ml // ¼ c red wine vinegar

SALAD

- 🍽 1 small head of iceberg lettuce
- 🍽 200g // 1c tomatoes, halved and quartered
- 🍽 1 small cucumber, peeled into ribbons
- 🍽 ½ red onion, finely sliced
- 🍽 180g // 1c black olives
- 🍽 150g // 1c feta, crumbled

DIRECTIONS

1. Begin by making your dressing. Do this by placing all ingredients into a small bowl and whisking until fully combined.
2. Assemble your salad by quartering your lettuce and arranging a quarter on each plate. Scatter your tomatoes around the lettuce, then arrange your cucumber ribbons, onion, and olives around the lettuce.

Drizzle your dressing over your salad before crumbling over your feta and serving.

Tuna Salad

Serves	4
Carbohydrates	8.1g
Protein	41g
Fat	10.1g
Calories	293

INGREDIENTS

TUNA

- 3 tbsp dark soy sauce
- 2 tbsp sesame oil
- 1 tsp rice wine vinegar
- 1 tsp olive oil
- 4 tuna steaks

SALAD

- 1 large cucumber, peel into ribbons
- 8 radish, finely sliced
- 2 sheets of nori, cut into thin strips
- 2 tbsp fresh ginger, minced
- 1 red chilli, deseeded and finely chopped
- 3 tbsp fresh coriander, finely chopped
- 2 tbsp fresh lime juice

DRESSING

- 4 tbsp full fat yoghurt
- 1 tsp dark soy sauce
- 1 tsp wasabi paste
- 4 tbsp fresh lime juice

DIRECTIONS

1. Pour your TUNA soy sauce, sesame oil, and rice wine vinegar into a shallow dish and whisk to combine before heating your olive oil in a large frying pan. Sear your tuna steaks for roughly 1 minute per side, or to your liking, then place into the marinade. Set the steaks aside for an hour, turning halfway through, to allow the flavours to fully infuse.

2. Whilst the tunas marinate tip all your SALAD ingredients into a large serving bowl. Toss everything together and set aside for 20-30 minutes to allow the flavours to infuse.

3. Once the steaks have marinated for an hour make your dressing by placing all DRESSING ingredients into a small bowl and whisking to fully combine. Divide your salad between 4 plates and slice the tuna before arranging it on top. Drizzle over a generous amount of dressing and serve.

Salmon Salad

Serves	4
Carbohydrates	7.7g
Protein	39.3g
Fat	23.5g
Calories	398

INGREDIENTS

- 1 lemon, zested and juiced
- 3 tbsp olive oil
- 2 tbsp full fat yoghurt
- 2 large courgettes, spiralised or peeled into ribbons
- 100g // 2/3 c fresh peas
- 4 radishes, thinly sliced
- 4 salmon fillets, poached and flaked
- Freshly ground black pepper
- 4 tbsp fresh dill, finely chopped, to serve
- 2 tbsp sunflower seeds to serve

DIRECTIONS

1. Make the dressing by whisking together your lemon juice, zest, yoghurt, and olive oil in a small bowl. Transfer your prepared courgettes, peas and radishes into a serving dish and toss everything together, before pouring over your dressing and tossing once again to ensure everything is coated.

Add half of your flaked salmon to the vegetables and toss to combine, then arrange the remainder of your salmon on top. Serve immediately with a grinding of pepper and sprinkling of dill and sunflower seeds, or divide between 4 plates before garnishing and serving.

Baked Cod

Serves	2
Carbohydrates	13g
Protein	30.5g
Fat	9.6g
Calories	266

INGREDIENTS

- 1 tsp olive oil
- 1 tbsp garlic, minced
- 1 shallot, sliced
- 200g // 7oz. fresh spinach
- 2 skinless cod fillets
- 50g // 2oz. goats cheese
- 4 plum tomatoes, sliced
- 2 sprigs of thyme to serve

DIRECTIONS

1. Begin by preheating your oven to 180C // 350F. Heat your oil over a medium heat in a large frying pan. Add your garlic and shallot and fry for 1-2 minutes, or until softened and aromatic, then add your spinach and heat briefly until it is wilted.

2. Spoon the wilted spinach into a small baking dish and arrange your cod fillets on top. Sprinkle over half of your goats cheese and arrange your tomatoes around the fillets, then transfer to the oven for 10-12 minutes, or until the fish is cooked and easily flakes.

Once cooked remove the fish from the oven. Divide the spinach and tomatoes between 2 plates before arranging your fillets on top. Sprinkle over your remaining goats cheese and top with your sprig of thyme to serve.

Shrimp and Grits

Serves	4
Carbohydrates	7.3g
Protein	37.6g
Fat	17.9g
Calories	365

INGREDIENTS

SHRIMP

- 2 tbsp garlic, minced
- 3 tsp smoked paprika
- 1 tsp cayenne pepper
- 2 tbsp butter, melted
- 450g // 1lb. shrimp, peeled and deveined

GRITS

- 1 tbsp butter
- 430g // 3c cauliflower rice
- 250ml // 1c full cream milk
- 90g // 1c grated parmesan
- Salt and pepper to taste
- Rocket to serve

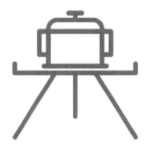

DIRECTIONS

1. Place your SHRIMP garlic, paprika, cayenne pepper, and 1 tbsp melted butter into a shallow dish and stir to combine. Pour in your prepared shrimp and toss the dish to ensure the shrimp are fully coated in the spices. Place the shrimp into the fridge and leave to marinate for at least 30 minutes.

2. While the shrimp marinate, heat your GRITS butter in a medium saucepan. Once melted pour in your cauliflower rice and heat for 2-3 minutes, or until the cauliflower has softened and absorbed the butter. Add in half or your milk and bring the mixture to the boil, then reduce the heat and leave to simmer for 5-10 minutes, or until the milk has been absorbed.

3. Once absorbed add in the remaining milk and stir to combine. Leave to simmer for a further 10 minutes, then stir in your grated parmesan and season with salt and pepper. Turn off the heat and set your grits aside.

In a large frying pan heat your remaining SHRIMP butter. Add in your marinated shrimp and cook over a medium heat for 3-5 minutes, or until cooked through. Ensure your grits are warm before serving with a side of rocket.

Saucy Chicken Meatballs

Serves	4
Carbohydrates	6.7g
Protein	35.9g
Fat	36.3g
Calories	498

INGREDIENTS

MEATBALLS

- 1 tbsp olive oil
- 1 small red onion
- 2 tbsp garlic, minced
- 450g // 1lb. ground chicken
- 4 tbsp fresh basil, finely chopped
- 1 tbsp Dijon mustard

SAUCE

- 400ml // 14oz. coconut milk
- 4 spring onions, finely sliced
- 1 tbsp garlic, minced
- Zest and juice of 1 lemon
- 6 tbsp fresh basil, finely chopped
- 1 tbsp mixed herbs
- Salt and pepper to taste
- Cauliflower rice or zoodles to serve

DIRECTIONS

1. Begin by preheating your oven to 180C // 350F and lining a large baking tray with foil or greaseproof paper.

2. Heat your oil in a large frying pan then add in your onion and garlic and cook for 3-5 minutes, or until softened and fragrant. Transfer your onion and garlic to a medium mixing bowl and leave to cool for 5-10 minutes before adding your chicken, basil, and mustard. Mix to combine everything with a wooden spoon or your hands, then shape into balls.

3. Arrange your meatballs on your prepared baking tray and transfer to the oven. Bake the meatballs for 15-20 minutes or until coloured and cooked through.

4. As your meatballs cook make your sauce by placing all your SAUCE ingredients into a food processor and blending until smooth and creamy. Transfer to a saucepan and heat.

Serve your meatballs hot with cauliflower rice or zoodles, topped with a generous serving of sauce.

Fried Chicken

Serves	4
Carbohydrates	4.3g
Protein	84.7g
Fat	70.3g
Calories	1008

INGREDIENTS

- 120g // 4oz. pork rinds
- 1 tsp chilli powder
- ½ tsp garlic powder
- 1 tsp smoked paprika
- ½ tsp oregano
- 1 tsp ground cumin
- Salt and pepper to taste
- 1 egg
- 60g // 2oz. mayonnaise
- 2 tbsp Dijon mustard
- 12 chicken thighs

DIRECTIONS

1. Begin by preheating your oven to 200C // 400F and lining a large baking tray with foil. Place your pork rinds, chilli, garlic powder, paprika, oregano, cumin, salt and pepper into a food processor. Pulse the mix to crush the pork rinds into irregularly sized pieces, then pour the mixture into a shallow dish.

2. In a large mixing bowl whisk together your egg, mayonnaise, and mustard. Place your chicken thighs in the bowl and toss to coat your chicken thighs in the egg mixture. One by one roll your chicken thighs in the pork rind mix and arrange on your prepared baking tray.

Once all your thighs have been 'breaded' transfer them to the oven and bake for 40-45 minutes, or until the chicken is cooked through and a crispy golden brown. Remove from the oven and serve immediately.

Chicken Stir Fry

Serves	4
Carbohydrates	6g
Protein	25.9g
Fat	9.8g
Calories	227

INGREDIENTS

- 2 tbsp sesame oil
- 4 spring onions, finely sliced
- 2 tbsp garlic, minced
- 1 red bell pepper, sliced
- 170g // 2c sugar snap peas
- 450g // 1lb. chicken breast, sliced into 1cm thick strips
- 3 tbsp dark soy sauce
- 2 tbsp rice wine vinegar
- 1 tbsp sriracha
- Salt and pepper to taste
- 2 tbsp sesame seeds to serve
- Fresh coriander to serve

DIRECTIONS

1. Heat your sesame oil in a wok over a medium heat. Add your spring onions and garlic and sauté for 1-2 minutes. Once the onions and garlic have softened add in your pepper and sugar snap peas to the wok and sauté for a further 3-5 minutes to soften.

2. Add your chicken to the vegetables and cook for 4-6 minutes, or until golden and cooked through, before adding your soy sauce, vinegar and sriracha. Toss to coat your chicken and vegetables in the liquid, then leave to simmer for 1-2 minutes.

Divide your stir fry between 4 bowls and top with sesame seeds and fresh coriander to serve.

Chicken Fritters

Serves	2
Carbohydrates	2.9g
Protein	32.2g
Fat	17.1g
Calories	302

INGREDIENTS

- 200g // 7oz. chicken breasts, cooked and shredded
- 1 egg
- 3 tsp mayonnaise
- 1 tsp chilli powder
- 1 red chilli, deseeded and finely sliced
- ½ tsp smoked paprika
- 1 tsp garlic, minced
- 2 tsp olive oil
- Leafy greens to serve

DIRECTIONS

1. Place your shredded chicken, egg, and mayonnaise in a medium mixing bowl. Stir to combine, then sprinkle over your chilli powder, red chilli, paprika, and garlic, and mix again to thoroughly combine.

2. Divide your mixture in 2 and shape each half into a thin patty. Place the patties in the fridge for 10 minutes to firm slightly. After 10 minutes remove your patties from the fridge and heat your oil in a medium frying pan.

Fry your patties for 3-4 minutes per side, making sure that each side becomes crispy and golden brown. Garnish your plate with leafy greens before arranging your patties on top and serving.

Chilli Bowls

Serves	4
Carbohydrates	6.7g
Protein	71.7g
Fat	17.4g
Calories	490

INGREDIENTS

- 2 tsp olive oil
- ½ small brown onion, sliced
- 4 tbsp tomato paste
- 1 tbsp chilli powder
- 1 tsp turmeric
- 3 tsp cumin
- 2 tsp smoked paprika
- 2 tbsp garlic, minced
- 60ml // ¼ c water
- 900g // 2lb. beef mince
- 280ml // 10oz. tinned tomatoes
- 500ml // 2c beef stock

DIRECTIONS

1. Heat your oil in a large heavy bottomed pan over a high heat, then add your onion, tomato paste, chilli powder, turmeric, cumin, paprika, and garlic. Sauté for 2-4 minutes, or until the onion is softened, then transfer to a food processor. Add in your water and blend until smooth.

2. Return your mix to your pan and heat to a boil, then reduce heat and leave to simmer for 3-5 minutes. Add in your beef mince, using a wooden spoon to break up the mince and combine with your blended spice mix.

3. Once the beef has started to brown pour in your tinned tomatoes and beef stock. Bring to the boil before reducing the heat and leaving the beef to simmer. Simmer for 30-40 minutes.

4. Serve the chilli once the liquid has reduced to a rich and meaty sauce.

Baked Pork Chops

Serves	6
Carbohydrates	1.2g
Protein	18.2g
Fat	20g
Calories	263

INGREDIENTS

- 1 tbsp cornflour
- ½ tsp salt
- 1 tsp paprika
- ½ tsp garlic powder
- ¼ tsp onion powder
- 1 tsp oregano
- 6 pork chops

DIRECTION

1. Begin by preheating your oven to 180C // 350F. In a medium bowl place your cornflour, salt, paprika, garlic powder, onion powder, and oregano. Stir to thoroughly combine.

2. Rinse your pork chops and dry with a paper towel, then place each chop into your herb mix. Toss the chop to fully coat in the seasoning before arranging on a large baking tray. Do this for all your chops.

3. Place your chops in the preheated oven and bake for 30-40 minutes or until the chops are golden brown and cooked through. Transfer to plates and serve immediately.

Smoked Pork Tenderloin

Serves	4
Carbohydrates	1.1g
Protein	30.3g
Fat	8.2g
Calories	206

INGREDIENTS

- 450g // 1lb. pork tenderloin
- 60ml // ¼ c Dijon mustard
- 1 tbsp garlic, minced
- 1 tsp chilli powder
- 1 tsp oregano
- 1 tsp mixed herb
- Salt and pepper to taste
- 1 tbsp olive oil
- Hickory wood chips

DIRECTIONS

1. Prepare your pork by trimming away any excess fat and skin, then massage your mustard and garlic into your pork. Mix your chilli powder, oregano, mixed herbs, salt and pepper in a small bowl, then sprinkle over your pork. Massage your herbs into your pork.

2. Wrap your pork tightly in clingfilm and leave in the fridge for at least 2 hours, preferably overnight. When you are ready to cook your pork remove it from the fridge 30 minutes prior to cooking to allow it to heat to room temperature.

3. Place a layer of wood chips into your barbeque and scatter charcoal briquettes on top. Light your briquettes and place the lid over your barbeque to keep in the smoke. While the wood chips begin to smoke heat your oil in a medium frying pan and sear your pork tenderloin all over.

4. Place your seared pork into the barbeque and replace the lid. Cook the pork for 2-2.5 hours, checking every 30 minutes that the briquettes are still warm, and the wood chips are smoking- both will most likely need to be replenished during the cooking process.

Once your pork is cooked through remove it from the barbeque and set aside to rest for 5-10 minutes. Slice your tenderloin and serve while still warm.

Pizza Rolls

Serves	4
Carbohydrates	4.5g
Protein	16.5g
Fat	16.9g
Calories	241

INGREDIENTS

DOUGH

-  350g // 12oz. grated mozzarella
- 2 tbsp cream cheese
- 90g // ¾ c almond flour
- 1 egg
- 2 tsp garlic, minced

FILLING

- 2 tbsp marinara sauce
- 225g // 8oz. grated mozzarella
- Extra topping – olives, peppers, salami, bacon, etc.

DIRECTIONS

1. Begin by preheating your oven to 200C // 400F and lining a baking tray with greaseproof paper. Melt your DOUGH mozzarella in the microwave at 20 second intervals until fully melted- this should take roughly 1 minute. Stir in your cream cheese and heat in the microwave for a further 20 seconds.

2. Pour your almond flour, egg, and garlic into your melted cheese mixture and stir to thoroughly combine. Once combined transfer the dough to your prepared baking tray and flatten into a large rectangle.

3. Transfer your dough to the oven and bake for 5 minutes. After 5 minutes remove your dough from the oven. Spread over your marinara sauce and sprinkle over your FILLING mozzarella- add any extra toppings at this point, ensuring everything is evenly distributed.

4. Starting at one of the longer edges lift your greaseproof paper and roll your pizza up into a log. Use a serrated knife to cut the log into 1cm thick rounds, then arrange these back on your baking tray.

Return your prepared pizza rolls to the oven and bake for a further 10-15 minutes, or until the dough is golden brown and the cheese inside is melted. Remove from the oven and serve immediately.

Lasagne

Serves	4
Carbohydrates	13.1g
Protein	36g
Fat	21.5g
Calories	396

INGREDIENTS

- 1 large courgette, peeled into strips
- 2 tbsp olive oil
- 450g // 16oz. beef mince
- 1 tbsp garlic, minced
- 250ml // 1c marinara sauce
- 280g // 10oz. ricotta cheese
- 110g // 4oz. grated mozzarella
- Salt and pepper to taste

DIRECTIONS

1. Begin by preheating your oven to 180C // 350F. Prepare your courgette by peeling it into strips- these will substitute the lasagne sheets. Sprinkle salt over the strips and leave them on a paper towel for 15-20 minutes to absorb any excess moisture.

2. While your courgette rests heat your oil in a large pan. Add in your beef mince and garlic and cook for 5 minutes, or until the beef is broken up and browned. Season with salt and pepper before pouring in your marinara sauce and stirring to combine.

3. Assemble your lasagne in a small baking dish. Layer the ingredients in the following order:

4. beef – ricotta – courgette – beef – ricotta – courgette – beef – ricotta – mozzarella.

Cover your lasagne with foil and transfer to your preheated oven. Bake for 30-40 minutes before removing the foil and allowing the cheese to melt and crisp for a further 5 minutes. Remove from the oven and serve immediately.

Falafel Wraps

Serves	4
Carbohydrates	13.3g
Protein	44.1g
Fat	54.8g
Calories	724

INGREDIENTS

- 🍽 75g // ½ c sliced almonds
- 🍽 75g // ½ c pumpkin seeds
- 🍽 225g // 3c mushrooms sliced
- 🍽 125ml // ½ c olive oil
- 🍽 175ml // ¾ c pea protein powder
- 🍽 4tbsp chia seeds
- 🍽 1 tbsp diced garlic
- 🍽 1 tbsp coriander finely chopped
- 🍽 1 tsp ground cumin
- 🍽 1 tsp turmeric
- 🍽 1 tbsp onion powder
- 🍽 60ml // ¼ c water
- 🍽 4 large lettuce, cabbage, or kale leaves
- 🍽 Salt and pepper to taste

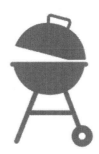

DIRECTIONS

1. Begin by preheating your oven to 180C // 350F and greasing a baking sheet. Toast almonds and pumpkin seeds in an unoiled frying pan for 2 minutes, then transfer to a food processor and pulse until they are finely chopped, but still have texture.

2. Sautee mushrooms and garlic in 1 tbsp of the oil until soft, then transfer them and the remaining ingredients to the food processor. Blend once again, before pouring everything into a large bowl, and mixing by hand to ensure everything is fully combined.

Divide the mixture into 4 before shaping each portion into 3 balls or sausages. Bake in the preheated oven for 15-20 minutes, or until golden and crispy. Remove them from the oven and serve each portion inside a leaf to create a falafel wrap.

EXCLUSIVE BONUS

40 Weight Loss Recipes

&

14 Days Meal Plan

Scan the QR-Code and receive
the FREE download:

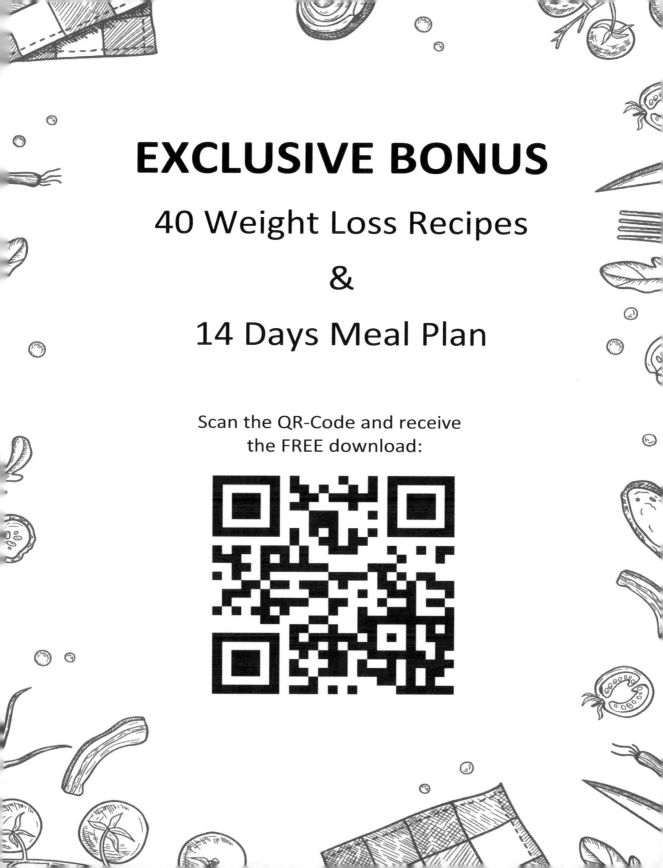

30 DAYS DIET PLAN

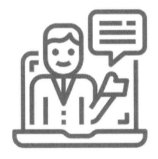

Day 1

Breakfast: Berry Blast Smoothie (See page 24)

Lunch: Salmon Salad (See page 40)

Dinner: Sausage and Mushroom Frittata

Serves	4
Carbohydrates	1.1g
Protein	26.2g
Fat	30.1g
Calories	384

INGREDIENTS

- 75g // 2.5oz. sliced mushrooms
- 300g // 10.5oz. sausage, chopped
- 8 eggs
- 1 tbsp garlic, minced
- Salt and pepper to taste

DIRECTIONS

1. Begin by preheating your oven to 200C // 400F and oiling a large baking dish. Fry your garlic, mushrooms, and sausage in a large pan until cooked and crispy, then transfer to the oiled dish.

2. In a separate bowl whisk eggs until foamy, adding the salt and pepper for taste. Pour the eggs over the fried ingredients in the dish before transferring it to the preheated oven.

Bake in the centre of the oven for 15-20 minutes. After this time has passed turn the oven off but leave the door ajar to rest the frittata for 5 minutes prior to removal and serving.

Day 2

Breakfast: Keto Bread

Serves	1
Carbohydrates	6g
Protein	8.6g
Fat	21.5g
Calories	269

INGREDIENTS

- 1 egg
- 1 tbsp milk
- 1 tbsp olive oil
- 1 tbsp coconut flour
- 1 tbsp almond flour
- ¼ tsp baking powder
- Pinch of salt

DIRECTIONS

1. Whisk together the egg, milk, and oil. Add in your flours, baking powder, and salt, and stir to combine.
2. Pour mix into a microwave safe mug, allowing the mixture room to rise, then microwave on high for 1 minute 30 seconds.

TO TOAST

1. Remove your bread from the mug and cut into 1-1.5 cm slices.
2. Fry the slices in a small, oiled pan, turning until both sides are browned and crispy.

Lunch: Gazpacho (See page 33)

Dinner: Chicken Stir Fry (See page 47)

Day 3

Breakfast: Mushroom Baked Eggs (See page 10)

Lunch: Chicken Fajita Bowl

Serves	4
Carbohydrates	14.1g
Protein	33.2g
Fat	23.3g
Calories	419

INGREDIENTS

- 1 head romaine lettuce
- 10 cherry tomatoes
- 1 avocado
- 2 tbsp finely chopped coriander
- 1/2 yellow onion
- 1/2 green pepper
- 325g // 11oz. chicken thighs
- 1 tbsp taco spice or tex-mex seasoning
- Salt and pepper to taste
- 75g // 1c grated cheddar
- 125ml // ½ c sour cream

DIRECTIONS

1. Prepare your base by chopping lettuce, tomatoes, avocado, and dividing between 2 bowls.
2. Cut the chicken into thin strips and fry in a medium pan with oil, salt, and pepper.
3. Whilst the chicken fries, finely slice the onion and pepper. When the chicken is almost cooked through add the onion, pepper, and seasoning whilst stirring.
4. Turn the heat to low and allow to cook for a few more minutes, before transferring the mixture to your prepared bowls. Top with the shredded cheese and sour cream to serve.

Dinner: Lasagne (See page 55)

Day 4

Breakfast: Pumpkin Pancakes (See page 22)

Lunch: Celery Soup (See page 29)

Dinner: Bolognaise

Serves	4
Carbohydrates	7.3g
Protein	36.3g
Fat	10.9g
Calories	284

INGREDIENTS

BOLOGNAISE

- 1/2 yellow onion, diced
- 2 tbsp garlic minced
- 2 celery stalks, each about 20cm long
- 450g // 1lb. beef mince
- 1 heaped tbsp tomato puree
- 2 tsp Worcester sauce
- 1 tsp dried oregano
- 1 tsp dried basil
- Salt and pepper to taste

ZOODLES

- 3 medium courgettes
- 1 tbsp olive oil

DIRECTIONS

1. Sautee finely chopped onion, garlic, and celery in a large pan on a high heat. Once browned and softened add the remaining ingredients and seasoning, making sure to stir and combine.

2. Simmer on a low heat for at least 30 minutes, stirring regularly. If the sauce seems too thick at this point at 1tbsp of water and stir.

3. Whilst the beef mixture simmers make your zoodles by using a spiralizer, mandolin, or peeler to cut courgette into ribbons. Alternatively, you can buy pre-spiralized courgette.

4. Heat the oil in a frying pan and flash fry the zoodles so they are softened but maintaining some crunch.

Transfer zoodles to a bowl, then top with the bolognaise and serve.

Day 5

Breakfast: Lemon and Blueberry Muffins

Serves	12
Carbohydrates	2.8g
Protein	5.3g
Fat	17.2g
Calories	193

INGREDIENTS

- 360g // 3c almond flour
- 120ml // ½ c melted butter
- 3 eggs
- 1 tbsp lemon zest
- 1 tsp vanilla extract
- 50g // ¼ c sweetener, such as stevia or swerve
- 1 tsp baking powder
- ¼ tsp salt
- 50g // 1/3 c blueberries
- 2 tbsp lemon juice
- Extra lemon zest to serve

DIRECTIONS

1. Begin by preheating your oven to 180C // 350F and line a 12-hole muffin or cupcake tray.

2. Place your flour, melted butter, eggs, lemon zest, vanilla extract, sweetener, baking powder, and salt into a large bowl. Using a wooden spoon or handheld mixer beat everything together until it has formed a thick batter. Gently mix in your blueberries, using a wooden spoon to avoid bursting or crushing them.

3. Divide the batter equally between your 12 lined holes before placing into the centre of your preheated oven. Bake for 15-20 minutes, or until firm and with some colour, checking they are done by pricking with a skewer that will come out clean.

4. Remove the muffins from the oven and leave to cool slightly before brushing with lemon juice and decorating with more lemon zest.

Lunch: Chilli Bowls (See page 49)
Dinner: Chicken Fritters (See page 48)

Day 6

Breakfast: Bacon Breakfast Tacos (See page 14)

Lunch: Cheesy Chips

Serves	4
Carbohydrates	4g
Protein	2.2g
Fat	13.8g
Calories	147

INGREDIENTS

- 2 medium turnips
- ½ tsp garlic powder
- ½ tsp smoked paprika
- Salt and pepper to taste
- 3 tbsp olive oil
- 60g // ½ c grated mozzarella
- 4 tbsp sour cream
- Green onions to garnish

DIRECTIONS

1. Begin by preheating your oven to 200C // 400F. Peel your turnips and slice into 1cm thick 'fries'.

2. Transfer turnips to a baking tray and add the garlic powder, paprika, seasoning, and oil, then toss it all together to ensure the fries are evenly coated. Roast in the preheated oven for 35-40 minutes, or until cooked through, golden, and crispy.

3. Top the fries with your grated mozzarella (and any extras you may wish to add) before returning to the oven for a further 5 minutes to melt the cheese.

4. Transfer to plates and serve with a spoon of sour cream and sprinkling of green onions.

Dinner: Shrimp and Grits (See page 42)

Day 7

Breakfast: Egg and Feta Hash (See page 13)
Lunch: Mushroom Soup (See page 28)
Dinner: Butter Chicken

Serves	4
Carbohydrates	5.1g
Protein	66.1g
Fat	28.5g
Calories	558

INGREDIENTS

SAUCE

- 1 tomato chopped
- 1 yellow onion chopped
- 2 tbsp freshly grated ginger
- 2 garlic cloves minced
- 1 tbsp tomato paste

- 1 tbsp garam masala spice
- 1 tsp chilli flakes
- 1 tsp salt
- 175ml // ¾ c heavy whipping cream

CHICKEN

- 900g // 2lb. boneless chicken thighs cut into bite sized pieces
- 4 tbsp butter
- Sliced coriander to serve

DIRECTIONS

1. Create the sauce by placing all ingredients, except the cream, into a food processor and blending until a smooth paste is formed. Add the cream to this paste and blend once again until fully combined.

2. Place your chopped chicken into a large bowl and pour the sauce over, stirring to ensure all chicken is covered. Leave this to marinate in the fridge for at least 30 minutes.

3. After 30 minutes or more, remove the chicken from the sauce and heat 2tbsp of butter in a pan. Fry the chicken for 4-6 minutes, before pouring over the remaining sauce and the remaining tbsp of butter. Turn the heat to low so the mixture can simmer for around 15 minutes, or until the chicken is cooked through.

Add salt to taste before garnishing with coriander and serving.

Day 8

Breakfast: Everything Bagels (See page 17)

Lunch: Cauliflower Cheese

Serves	4
Carbohydrates	5g
Protein	12g
Fat	17.2g
Calories	226

INGREDIENTS

- 450g // 1lb. cauliflower florets
- 120ml // ½ c sour cream
- 1 tsp smoked paprika
- 1 tsp garlic powder
- 3 tbsp butter
- 110g // ½ c grated mozzarella
- 110g // ½ c grated cheddar
- 1 tsp fresh chilli, sliced
- Salt and pepper to taste
- Extra chilli to serve

DIRECTIONS

1. Begin by preheating your oven to 200C // 400F. Bring a large saucepan of salted water to the boil and boil your cauliflower for 5-10 minutes, or until cooked and softened. Drain the water and leave your cauliflower to cool for a couple of minutes, then transfer to a kitchen towel or cheesecloth and firmly squeeze out any excess liquid.

2. Place your cauliflower, sour cream, paprika, garlic powder, and butter in a food processor. Blend until everything is combined and the cauliflower mix resembles mashed potatoes. Transfer the mix to a baking dish and stir in your sliced chilli and half of your grated cheeses.

3. Sprinkle over the remaining half of your grated cheeses and season with salt and pepper, then transfer to your preheated oven. Bake for 5-10 minutes, or until the cheese is melted and bubbling. If you want your cheese to go crispy bake for a further 5 minutes.

4. Remove your cauliflower cheese from the oven and sprinkle over a little extra sliced chilli to garnish, then serve immediately.

Dinner: Baked Cod (See page 41)

Day 9

Breakfast: Egg and Ham Wrap (See page 20)
Lunch: Goats Cheese and Celery Boats (See page 36)
Dinner: Grilled Salmon

Serves	4
Carbohydrates	3.9g
Protein	35.4g
Fat	11.2g
Calories	255

INGREDIENTS

- 4 salmon fillets
- 1 lemon
- 2 tbsp garlic, minced
- 1 tbsp fresh rosemary, finely chopped
- 1 tbsp fresh thyme, finely chopped
- 1 shallot, finely chopped
- 1 tbsp Dijon mustard
- Salt and pepper to taste

DIRECTIONS

1. Start by setting your grill to medium and leaving it to heat, then line a medium baking tray with parchment paper and arrange your salmon fillets on top.
2. Place your garlic, rosemary, thyme, shallot, and mustard in a small bowl. Halve your lemon and squeeze in the juice from one half, then stir everything together before seasoning with salt and pepper and stirring again.

Brush the mixture over the fillets, then place them under the grill for 6-8 minutes, or until pink and cooked. Once cooked transfer the salmon to serving plates. Cut your remaining lemon half into quarters, and serve each fillet with a slice of lemon.

Day 10

Breakfast: Breakfast Bars

Serves	6
Carbohydrates	5.7g
Protein	3.6g
Fat	26.1g
Calories	268

INGREDIENTS

- 🍽 60g // ½ c cashew nuts
- 🍽 120g // ½ c cashew butter
- 🍽 60ml // ¼ c coconut oil
- 🍽 6 tbsp desiccated coconut
- 🍽 50g // ¼ c sweetener, such as stevia or swerve

DIRECTIONS

1. Begin by lining a small baking tin with parchment paper. Place your cashew nuts into a food processor and pulse on high until they are crushed but retaining some texture. Alternatively crush them by hand by placing the nuts into a Ziploc bag and gently hitting with a rolling pin.

2. Pour your cashew butter, coconut oil, and desiccated coconut into a medium mixing bowl and stir to thoroughly combine. Add your crushed nuts and sweetener before stirring again until a thick batter has formed.

3. Pour the batter into the prepared baking tin and use the back of a spoon to spread the mixture evenly, ensuring that all corners of the tin are filled.

4. Chill in the fridge for at least an hour (preferably overnight) before cutting into 6 and serving.

Lunch: Clam Chowder (See page 31)
Dinner: Pizza Rolls (See page 53)

Day 11

Breakfast: Stuffed Tomatoes (See page 19)
Lunch: Fried Chicken (See page 46)
Dinner: Baked Brie

Serves	4
Carbohydrates	2.8g
Protein	6.9g
Fat	18.2g
Calories	206

INGREDIENTS

- 1 medium brie wheel
- 1 tbsp olive oil
- 1 small yellow onion, sliced
- 2 tbsp balsamic vinegar
- 2 tbsp garlic, minced
- 1 tbsp olive oil
- 2 tbsp fresh rosemary, chopped
- 3 tbsp walnuts, finely chopped

DIRECTIONS

1. Begin by preheating your oven to 200C // 400F and lining a small baking tray with parchment paper.

2. Heat your olive oil in a small frying pan over a medium heat. Once hot, pour in your sliced onions, balsamic vinegar, and 2 tbsp of water. Cover the pan and sauté the onions for 2-4 minutes, shaking the pan to ensure the onions don't burn. Once softened remove from the heat and set aside.

3. Place your garlic, olive oil, and rosemary in a small bowl. Heat in the microwave for 2 seconds, then remove from the microwave and add in your finely chopped walnuts and stirring to ensure the walnuts are coated.

4. Place your brie wheel onto the prepared baking tray. Take a sharp knife and make a few small scores all over the cheese. Place your sauteed onions in the centre of the cheese, then pour over your oil and nut mix.

Transfer the baking tray to the preheated oven and bake the cheese for 10-15 minutes, or until the cheese is warm and aromatic. Remove from the oven and serve immediately.

Day 12

Breakfast: Savoury Cauliflower Waffles (See page 21)

Lunch: Shrimp Skewers

Serves	4
Carbohydrates	3.6g
Protein	21.6g
Fat	8.9g
Calories	176

INGREDIENTS

- 450g // 1lb. large shrimps
- 3 tbsp butter, melted
- 2 tbsp harissa paste
- 1 tsp cayenne pepper
- 1 tsp ground cumin
- 1 tbsp fresh lime juice
- 2 tbsp garlic, minced
- Salt and pepper to taste
- 1 lime, quartered
- 1 tbsp fresh coriander, finely chopped

DIRECTIONS

1. Begin by peeling and deveining your shrimp. After doing this season them with salt and pepper and set aside.

2. In a medium bowl mix together your melted butter, harissa paste, cayenne pepper, cumin, lime juice, and garlic. Season with salt and pepper, then pour in your shrimp. Toss the shrimp to ensure all are evenly covered, and preferably leave to marinade for at least 30 minutes.

3. After the shrimp have marinated, divide them equally between 4 skewers, leaving a small gap between each shrimp on the skewer.

4. Place a large frying pan over a high heat. Once the pan is hot, add the skewers, cooking for 2-3 minutes on each side, or until fully cooked through.

5. Transfer the skewers to plates and serve finished with a lime wedge and a sprinkling of coriander.

Dinner: Baked Pork Chops (See page 50)

Day 13

Breakfast: Cauliflower Toast

Serves	2
Carbohydrates	8.4g
Protein	10.4g
Fat	3.8g
Calories	124

INGREDIENTS

- 1 medium cauliflower head
- 1 large egg
- 40g // ½ c grated mozzarella
- ½ tbsp garlic powder
- Salt and pepper to taste

DIRECTIONS

1. Begin by preheating your oven to 200C // 400 F and greasing or lining a large baking tray.
2. Break your cauliflower into florets and place these into a food processor. Pulse on high until your cauliflower is fully broken down and has a grainy, sand-like texture. Transfer the cauliflower into a large microwave proof bowl and heat on high for 7 minutes. Once heated pour your mixture into a tea towel or cheesecloth and squeeze firmly to remove any excess moisture.
3. Pour your cauliflower back into your bowl and add in the egg, mozzarella, garlic powder, and salt and pepper to season. Use your hands or a wooden spoon to thoroughly combine everything.
4. Divide your mixture into 6. Place each portion onto your prepared baking tray and shape to resemble a slice of toast. Transfer the tray into your preheated oven and bake for 12-15 minutes, or until the 'toast' is golden and crispy.
5. Remove from the oven and serve immediately, topping with eggs, bacon, avocado, cheese, or anything else.

Lunch: Greek Salad Slabs (See page 37)

Dinner: Saucy Chicken Meatballs (See page 44)

Day 14

Breakfast: Granola (See page 25)

Lunch: Cauliflower Steak (See page 35)

Dinner: Zoodle Alfredo

Serves	4
Carbohydrates	9.1g
Protein	9.6g
Fat	40.8g
Calories	447

INGREDIENTS

- 🍽 2 tsp olive oil
- 🍽 1 shallot, chopped
- 🍽 3 tbsp garlic, minced
- 🍽 60ml // ¼ c white wine
- 🍽 370ml // 1 ½ c double cream
- 🍽 2 dried bay leaves
- 🍽 60g // ½ c grated parmesan
- 🍽 450g // 1lb. zoodles
- 🍽 Salt and pepper to taste

DIRECTIONS

1. Heat your oil in a large frying pan. Add your shallots and minced garlic, then cook until softened and aromatic- roughly 3 minutes. Pour in your white wine and leave to simmer.

2. Once the wine has reduced by roughly half pour in your double cream and bay leaves. Bring the mixture to a boil and stir continuously until the sauce begins to thicken. Reduce the heat to low and pour in your grated parmesan, then season with salt and pepper, stirring until the parmesan has melted into the sauce.

Remove the bay leaves from the sauce before adding in the zoodles. Toss the zoodles in the sauce so they are fully coated, then remove the pan from the heat. Serve the dish warm, topping with additional grated parmesan and a generous sprinkling of cracked black pepper.

Day 15

Breakfast: Egg and Bacon Avocado Boats

Serves	4
Carbohydrates	4.5g
Protein	26.6g
Fat	54.4g
Calories	641

INGREDIENTS

- 4 ripe avocados
- 8 medium eggs
- 6 bacon rashers
- Chilli flakes to taste
- Salt and pepper to season

DIRECTIONS

1. Begin by preheating your oven to 180C // 350F. Prepare your avocados by halving and stoning each, and then scooping out some flesh from each half so that the remaining flesh is left as a 1cm border.

2. Place your prepared avocados into a large baking dish and crack an egg into each of the hollows. Season with salt and pepper, and sprinkle over your chilli flakes, before placing into the preheated oven.

3. As your avocados cook dice your bacon rashers and place them into a large, oiled frying pan over a high heat. Fry your bacon until crisp and browned before transferring onto a paper towel lined plate.

4. After 15-20 minutes your avocados should be cooked- the whites should be firm, and the yolks should still be runny. Remove them from the oven and transfer to plates. Sprinkle over your crispy bacon and serve.

Lunch: Tuna Salad (See page 38)

Dinner: Smoked Pork Tenderloin (See page 51)

Day 16

Breakfast: Egg and Asparagus Soldiers (See page 12)

Lunch: Chicken Nuggets

Serves	4
Carbohydrates	9.9g
Protein	44.6g
Fat	29.3g
Calories	487

INGREDIENTS

- 500g // 1.1lb. boneless chicken breast or thighs, cut into bite sized pieces
- 75g // 1/2c shredded parmesan cheese
- ½ tsp onion powder
- 1 egg
- Salt and pepper to taste
- 2 tsp coconut oil

BEAN FRIES

- 150g // 1c green beans trimmed
- 2 tsp coconut oil

BBQ DIPPING SAUCE

- 125ml // 2/3c mayonnaise
- 2 tsp tomato puree
- ½ tsp smoked paprika
- ½ tsp garlic powder
- Salt and pepper to taste

DIRECTIONS

1. Begin by preheating your oven to 180C // 350F and oiling a medium baking tray. Create the nugget crumb by thoroughly combining the parmesan and onion powder in a medium mixing bowl. In a separate bowl whisk the egg until frothy, adding salt and pepper to season.

2. Mix your chicken pieces into the egg and make sure that they are evenly coated with egg mixture. One at a time remove your chicken pieces from the egg mixture and coat in the nugget crumb, before shaking off any excess and placing evenly spaced on the baking tray. Repeat until all the chicken is used up.

3. Bake the chicken in the oven for 15-20 minutes, or until crispy and cooked through. Turn halfway through baking.

4. Whilst the chicken is baking make the bean fries by heating the oil in a medium pan over a high heat. Once the oil is melted add the beans and fry for a few minutes so they are crispy- if fried for too long they will soften and wilt.

5. Make the dipping sauce by combining all the ingredients in a small bowl, adjusting spice measurements to taste. Once the chicken is cooked transfer to plates and serve with the bean fries and BBQ dipping sauce.

Dinner: Slow Cooker Prawn Soup (See page 30)

Day 17

Breakfast: Cauliflower Eggs Benedict (See page 15)

Lunch: Chicken Stir Fry (See page 47)

Dinner: Mediterranean Fish Traybake

Serves	2
Carbohydrates	14.3g
Protein	42g
Fat	33.6g
Calories	531

INGREDIENTS

- 3 tbsp harissa paste
- 1 lemon
- 2 tbsp olive oil
- 2 white fish fillets (cod and haddock work best)
- 1 medium courgette
- 1 yellow pepper
- 1 red pepper
- ½ red onion
- 30g // ¼ c pitted black olives
- 2 tbsp toasted pine nuts

DIRECTIONS

1. Begin by preheating your oven to 200C // 400F. Create the marinade by mixing the harissa paste, juice of ½ the lemon, a pinch of salt, and 2 tbsp of olive oil. Combine until it forms a loose paste.

2. Use half of the marinade to coat your fish fillets, then set them aside to absorb the flavours. Chop the peppers, courgette, olives, and onion into slices, before placing into a roasting dish and tossing with the remaining marinade.

3. Slice the remaining ½ of your lemon into 0.5cm rounds and place on top of your vegetable mixture. Roast the veg for 15-20 minutes before placing the fish on top and cooking for a further 12-15 mins. The remaining cooking time is dependent upon the thickness of your fish fillets.

Remove from the oven and serve immediately, topping with toasted pine nuts.

Day 18

Breakfast: Lemon and Blueberry Muffins (See page 65)

Lunch: Thai Butternut Soup (See page 34)

Dinner: Broccoli and Parmesan Fritters

Serves	4
Carbohydrates	5.2g
Protein	12.8g
Fat	12.7g
Calories	189

INGREDIENTS

- 🍽 350g // 1 medium broccoli head
- 🍽 4 eggs
- 🍽 35g // 1/3 c almond flour
- 🍽 50g // ½ c grated parmesan
- 🍽 1 tsp onion powder
- 🍽 1 tbsp garlic, minced
- 🍽 1 tsp chilli flakes
- 🍽 Salt and pepper to taste
- 🍽 1 tbsp butter
- 🍽 Chilli flakes to serve

DIRECTIONS

1. Chop the broccoli into florets before placing them into a food processor. Pulse until the broccoli is finely chopped to a sand like consistency.

2. Pour the blended broccoli onto a dishtowel or kitchen paper and leave for 10 minutes to remove any excess moisture.

3. After the 10 minutes add all your ingredients in a large mixing bowl and stir thoroughly to ensure everything is combined. Leave to stand for a further 10 minutes before stirring once again. Divide the mixture into 4 and shape each ¼ into a fritter.

Heat your oil in a large non-stick pan. Fry the fritters for about 4 minutes per side, making sure the bottom is cooked and crisp before flipping. Once cooked through transfer to a paper towel lined plate. Once all the fritters are cooked serve them warm and with a sprinkling of chilli flakes.

Day 19

Breakfast: Green Smoothie

Serves	1
Carbohydrates	6g
Protein	7.6g
Fat	27.9g
Calories	307

INGREDIENTS

- 75ml // 1/3 c coconut milk
- 150ml // 2/3 c water
- 2 tbsp lime juice
- 170g // ¾ c spinach
- 1 tbsp fresh ginger, grated
- 1 tsp desiccated coconut to serve

DIRECTIONS

1. Place coconut milk, water, and spinach into blender and liquidise.
2. Add lime juice and ginger to taste.
3. Serve cold with a lime wedge and a sprinkle of desiccated coconut.

Lunch: Cauliflower Cheese (See page 70)

Dinner: Falafel Wraps (See page 57)

Day 20

Breakfast: Granola (See page 25)

Lunch: Turkey Stir Fry

Serves	4
Carbohydrates	2.5g
Protein	28.4g
Fat	8.6g
Calories	195

INGREDIENTS

- 450g // 1lb. turkey tenderloin, cut into 1cm slices
- 1 small onion, sliced
- 1 red bell pepper, sliced
- 1 yellow bell pepper, sliced
- 2 tbsp olive oil
- 1 tsp mixed herbs
- 1 tbsp red wine vinegar
- 125ml // ½ c tinned tomatoes
- Salt and pepper to taste

DIRECTIONS

1. Heat your oil in a large pan and add in your sliced turkey. Cook for 2-5 minutes, browning both sides and cooking through.
2. Add in your onion and peppers, then season with salt and pepper. Cover the pan with a lid and sauté on low for 5-7 minutes, or until the vegetables are softened and starting to brown- be sure to remove the lid and stir every couple of minutes.
3. Increase the heat to medium and add in your mixed herbs, vinegar, and tinned tomatoes. Stir everything together and leave to simmer for 5 minutes, or until the sauce has reduced by ¼ - ½.
4. Ensure the turkey is hot before serving.

Dinner: Sausage and Mushroom Frittata (See page 60)

Day 21

Breakfast: Berry Blast Smoothie (See page 24)

Lunch: Egg and Asparagus Soldiers (See page 12)

Dinner: Cashew Chicken

Serves	4
Carbohydrates	8.8g
Protein	14.1g
Fat	16.8g
Calories	245

INGREDIENTS

- 🍽 3 chicken thighs, boneless and deskinned
- 🍽 2 tbsp coconut oil
- 🍽 1 small white onion
- 🍽 1 small red pepper
- 🍽 ½ tsp fresh ginger, finely chopped
- 🍽 2 tbsp garlic, minced
- 🍽 1 tsp cayenne pepper
- 🍽 1 tbsp rice wine vinegar
- 🍽 1 tbsp soya sauce
- 🍽 40g // ¼ c cashew nuts
- 🍽 Salt and pepper to taste
- 🍽 1 tbsp sesame seeds
- 🍽 Sliced green onion

DIRECTIONS

1. Prepare your ingredients by cutting your chicken thighs into 1cm chunks and slicing your onion and pepper. Heat 1 tbsp of coconut oil in a large frying pan and add your chopped chicken thighs, cooking for 4-5 minutes, or until slightly brown and cooked through.

2. Increase the heat to high and add your remaining coconut oil to the pan, then pour in your onion, pepper, ginger, garlic, and cayenne pepper, and season with salt and pepper. Cook for another 2-3 minutes.

3. Add in your vinegar, soya sauce, and cashews, and toss everything together to ensure it is all coated with some sauce, then leave to cook down for 2-4 minutes.

Transfer to bowls and top with a sprinkling of sesame seed and green onion to serve.

Day 22

Breakfast: Bulletproof Coffee

Serves	1
Carbohydrates	0g
Protein	0.5g
Fat	36.7g
Calories	323

INGREDIENTS

- 1 cup of freshly brewed coffee
- 2 tbsp unsalted butter
- 1 tbsp coconut oil
- 1 tsp sweetener (if desired)
- A dash of milk (if desired)

DIRECTIONS

1. Pour all your ingredients into a food processor. Blend on high for 20-30 seconds, until the drink is aerated and frothy. Transfer to a mug and serve immediately, adding sweetener or milk to your liking.

Lunch: Shrimp and Grits (See page 42)
Dinner: Lasagne (See page 55)

Day 23

Breakfast: Cauliflower Toast (See page 78)

Lunch: Pumpkin and Feta Salad

Serves	2
Carbohydrates	10.9g
Protein	12.4g
Fat	44.4g
Calories	491

Ingredients

- 300g // 1 ½ c pumpkin cubed
- 150g // 1 c feta
- Leafy greens such as rocket, spinach, or romaine lettuce
- 4 tbsp olive oil
- 1 tbsp balsamic vinegar

DIRECTIONS

1. Before starting, preheat your oven to 200C // 400F.
2. Whilst the oven heats up peel and cube your pumpkin into bite sized pieces – the smaller your pieces the quicker the roasting time. Place these into a roasting tin and toss in 2tbsp of oil, plus salt and pepper to taste. Roast for 35-45 minutes, or until the pumpkin has darkened and softened.
3. Leave your pumpkin to cool, and in the meantime wash your leafy greens and mix the remaining 2 tbsp of olive oil with the balsamic to create a simple dressing
4. To serve layer the pumpkin on top of the greens and crumble the feta over. Drizzle with the balsamic dressing, and add pumpkin seeds or grated beetroot as an extra garnish if desired.

Dinner: Chicken Fajita Bowl (See page 62)

Day 24

Breakfast: Granola (See page 25)

Lunch: Mushroom Tacos

Serves	4
Carbohydrates	4.4g
Protein	2.8g
Fat	20.9g
Calories	222

INGREDIENTS

- 4 large portobello mushrooms, washed and with the stems removed
- 60g // ¼ c harissa paste
- 1 tsp ground cumin
- ½ tsp cayenne pepper
- 1 tsp onion powder
- 3 tbsp olive oil
- 1 large avocado, sliced
- 1 small red onion, diced
- 2 tbsp fresh coriander, chopped
- 4 large lettuce, cabbage, or kale leaves

DIRECTIONS

1. In a small bowl mix together your harissa paste, cumin, cayenne pepper, onion powder, and 1 ½ tbsp of olive oil until fully combined. Cover each mushroom in this harissa marinade and set aside for 10 minutes.

2. After 10 minutes heat your remaining oil in a large frying pan. Fry each mushroom for 2 minutes each side, or until slightly softened and browned. Remove the mushrooms from the heat and set aside.

3. Prepare your 'tacos' by putting a few slices of avocado along the stem of each leaf. Sprinkle over some of the diced red onion and some of the chopped coriander.

4. Slice each mushroom and place it in the prepared leaves. Serve your tacos topped with additional ingredients, for example salsa, cashew cream, or fresh chillies.

Dinner: Zoodle Alfredo (See page 80)

Day 25

Breakfast: Cinnamon Rolls

Serves	4
Carbohydrates	2.6g
Protein	9.8g
Fat	10g
Calories	139

INGREDIENTS

DOUGH

- 1 tbsp orange juice
- 340g // 1 ½ c grated mozzarella
- 2 tbsp cream cheese
- 1 egg
- 75g // ¾ c almond flour
- 1 tbsp sweetener, such as stevia or swerve

FILLING

- 1 tsp cinnamon
- 1 tsp nutmeg
- 1 tsp ginger
- 1 tbsp sweetener, such as stevia or swerve
- 2 tbsp warm water

ICING

- 1 tbsp cream cheese
- 1 tbsp Greek Yoghurt
- 1 tbsp sweetener, such as stevia or swerve

DIRECTIONS

1. Begin by preheating your oven to 180C // 350 F. To make the dough place your orange juice, grated mozzarella, and cream cheese into a large, microwave proof bowl, and heat on high for 20 second intervals until melted- this should take around 2 minutes.

2. Remove the mixture from the microwave and add in your egg, almond flour, and sweetener, stirring thoroughly to combine. Roll the dough out into a rectangle shape, placing it between two sheets of parchment paper to avoid sticking.

3. Transfer the dough to a large baking tray and place in the preheated oven for 5 minutes, before removing and setting aside to cool.

4. Whilst your dough cools mix together all your 'filling' ingredients in a small bowl. Spread this over your dough, being sure that all the dough is covered.

5. Starting from one of the long sides, roll your dough up to create one long log. Cut this into 4 thick rolls, then arrange on the baking tray and return to the oven. Bake for a further 5-7 minutes, or until firmed and golden.

6. Remove the rolls from the oven and leave to cool slightly. Whilst they cool make your icing, mixing together all 'icing' ingredients to form a thick paste. Spread this over the rolls and serve immediately whilst still warm.

Lunch: Celery Soup (See page 29)
Dinner: Chilli Bowls (See page 49)

Day 26

Breakfast: Herby Frittata (See page 11)

Lunch: Iceburgers

Serves	4
Carbohydrates	9.9g
Protein	54.8g
Fat	22.4g
Calories	475

INGREDIENTS

- 500g // 1.1lb. beef mince
- 1 tbsp mixed herbs
- 1 tbsp garlic, minced
- 1 tsp black pepper
- 1 tsp salt
- 1 tsp oil
- 4 bacon rashers
- 1 white or yellow onion, sliced
- 1 large head of iceberg lettuce
- 1 large tomato
- 4 slices of cheese, preferably cheddar or mozzarella

DIRECTIONS

1. Place your beef mince into a large bowl and add your mixed herbs, garlic, black pepper, and salt. Using your hands or a wooden spoon, mix everything together until thoroughly combined, then divide the mix into 4 and shape each portion into a burger patty, then set aside.

2. Heat 1tsp of oil in a large pan and fry your bacon until it is brown and crispy, then transfer to a paper towel lined plate. Using the same pan, turn the heat to medium and cook your burger patties. Cook the patties for about 4 minutes each side, or to your preference, the place a slice of cheese on each cooked burger. Turn off the heat and place a lid on the pan to melt the cheese.

3. Whilst the cheese melts, take your lettuce head and cut 8 rounds from your lettuce head to form 'buns', and cut your tomato into slices.

4. Assemble your burgers by placing a slice of tomato on the bottom 'bun'. Add your burger and a rasher of bacon, then top with another lettuce round 'bun'. Serve your burgers drizzled with ranch, tomato, or burger sauce.

Dinner: Mushroom Soup (See page 28)

Day 27

Breakfast: Oatmeal

Serves	1
Carbohydrates	5g
Protein	6g
Fat	32.9g
Calories	356

INGREDIENTS

- 110ml // ½ c coconut or almond milk (unsweetened)
- 2 tsp flaxseed
- 2 tsp chia seeds
- 1 tsp sunflower seeds
- Pinch of salt
- ½ tsp vanilla extract

DIRECTIONS

1. Heat the milk, sunflower seeds, flaxseed and chia in a small saucepan. Bring the mixture to a boil before turning the heat to medium and stirring in salt and vanilla extract to taste.

2. Keep the mixture on the heat, stirring occasionally, until your desired consistency is reached.

3. Transfer to a bowl and serve with a sprinkling of cinnamon, more seeds, or coconut cream.

Lunch: Greek Salad Slabs (See page 37)
Dinner: Smoked Pork Tenderloin (See page 51)

Day 28

Breakfast: Banana Waffles (See page 26)
Lunch: Pizza Rolls (See page 53)
Dinner: Pork Bowl

Serves	4
Carbohydrates	7.6g
Protein	32.9g
Fat	9.3g
Calories	260

INGREDIENTS

- 1 tbsp butter
- 2 tbsp garlic, minced
- 1 tbsp fresh ginger, finely chopped
- 1 small white onion, sliced
- 450g // 1lb. ground pork
- 1 medium carrot, grated
- ¼ small cabbage head, sliced
- 1 tbsp rice wine vinegar
- 1 tbsp siracha or chilli sauce
- 60ml // ¼ c soya sauce
- 2 tbsp peanuts, crushed

DIRECTIONS

1. Heat your butter in a large wok over a medium heat. Add your garlic and ginger, and sauté for 2 minutes, or until browning and aromatic. Add in your onion and sauté for a further 2-3 minutes, or until tender and translucent.

2. Add your ground pork to the wok, breaking it up to incorporate the other ingredients. Fry until all the pork is browned, then add in your carrot and cabbage, stirring everything until combined.

Pour in your vinegar, siracha, and soya sauce, and mix everything together. Cook for a further 5-7 minutes, or until the cabbage is wilted and tender, before dividing between 4 bowls and serving topped with crushed peanuts.

Day 29

Breakfast: Granola (See page 25)

Lunch: Cauliflower Steak (See page 35)

Dinner: Spinach and Artichoke Stuffed Chicken

Serves	4
Carbohydrates	2.4g
Protein	29.3g
Fat	20.6g
Calories	321

INGREDIENTS

- 4 large chicken breasts
- 80g // ½ c cream cheese
- 60ml // ¼ c Greek yoghurt
- 100g // 1/3 c grated mozzarella
- 4 marinated artichoke hearts, washed and roughly chopped
- 2 handfuls fresh spinach, shredded
- 1 tbsp mixed herbs
- 2 tbsp butter
- Salt and pepper to taste

DIRECTIONS

1. Score each chicken breast down the middle using a sharp knife. Carefully cut deeper on either side of the score to create a pocket for the filling, then take a rolling pin to tenderise the meat.

2. Combine your cream cheese, mozzarella, chopped artichoke hearts, shredded spinach, and mixed herbs in a large bowl. Season with salt and pepper, then mix thoroughly to ensure everything is combined.

3. Divide the filling between 4 and stuff each chicken breast with a portion of the cream cheese mixture. If necessary, take a couple of toothpicks and skewer the hole closed to avoid leakage.

Heat your butter in a large frying pan. Once melted add your stuffed chicken breasts to the pan, cooking each side for 5-7 minutes to ensure the chicken is golden brown, crispy, and cooked through, then transfer the stuffed breasts to plates and serve.

Day 30

Breakfast: Cloud Eggs

Serves	4
Carbohydrates	2.6g
Protein	30.4g
Fat	14.9g
Calories	268

INGREDIENTS

- 120g // 1c grated parmesan
- 250g // 9oz. cured ham, chopped
- 8 eggs whites
- 4 egg yolks
- Salt and pepper to taste
- Fresh basil to serve

DIRECTIONS

1. Start by preheating your oven to 200C // 450F and line a large baking tray with parchment paper, oil lightly oil it.

2. Have your egg whites in a large glass bowl, making sure the bowl is thoroughly cleaned beforehand, otherwise the whites will not whisk. Use a handheld whisk and beat the eggs on a high speed for 2-3 minutes, or until they double in size and form stiff white peaks.

3. Add your parmesan and ham to your egg whites then season with salt and pepper. Gently fold everything together, being sure to keep as much air in the whites as is possible.

4. Divide the mixture into 4 and spoon each portion onto the baking tray, leaving as much space as possible between them. Wet a serving spoon and press the back into each portion to create a small crater, then transfer to the preheated oven for 2-3 minutes.

5. Remove the baking try from the oven and place an egg yolk into each crater, then season again with salt and pepper. Return to the oven for a further 3-4 minutes, or until the whites are cooked through and slightly browned and the yolks have set slightly.

6. Transfer the eggs to plates and serve garnished with fresh basil.

Lunch: Gazpacho (See page 33)

Dinner: Salmon Salad (See page 40)

EXCLUSIVE BONUS

40 Weight Loss Recipes

&

14 Days Meal Plan

Scan the QR-Code and receive
the FREE download:

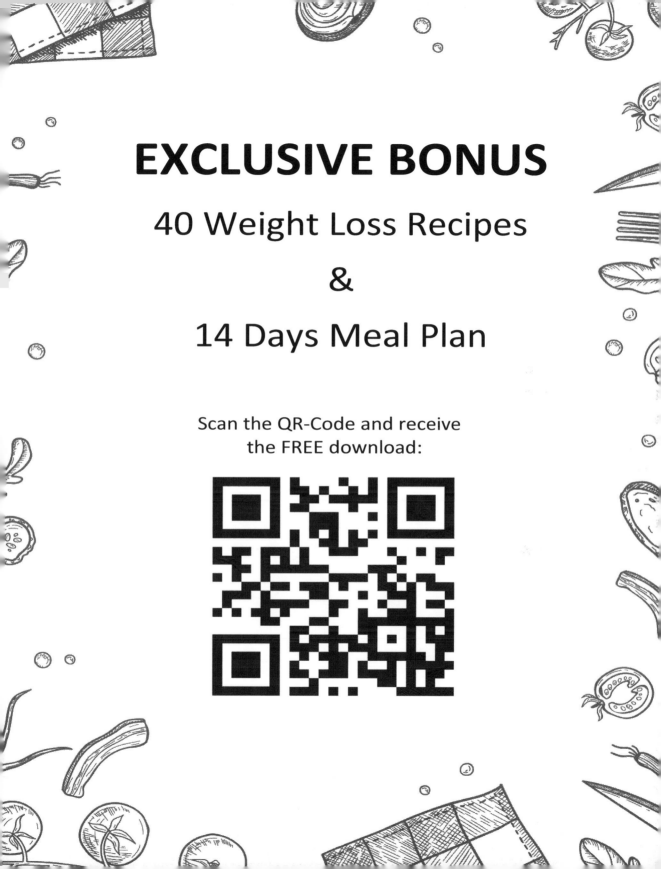

Disclaimer

This book contains opinions and ideas of the author and is meant to teach the reader informative and helpful knowledge while due care should be taken by the user in the application of the information provided. The instructions and strategies are possibly not right for every reader and there is no guarantee that they work for everyone. Using this book and implementing the information/recipes therein contained is explicitly your own responsibility and risk. This work with all its contents, does not guarantee correctness, completion, quality or correctness of the provided information. Misinformation or misprints cannot be completely eliminated.

Printed in Great Britain
by Amazon